Causes, Symptoms & Treatments

COPING WITH MENOPAUSE

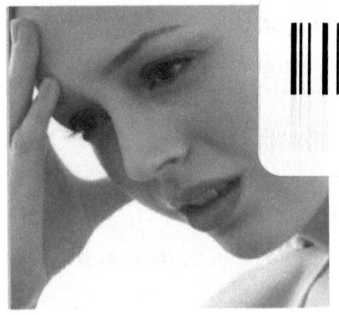

I0441543

Berna Vermont
Elsa Markeys
Susy Mora
Monica Parker
Daniel Parson

Vermont Indie Books

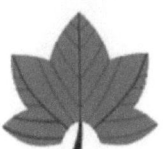

GRAPEVINE BOOKS
2015

DISCLAIMER

The duplication, sharing, uploading, transfer, and/or distribution of this electronic book by use of any digital, electronic, or printed process without the explicit permission of the publisher is unauthorized. These pages are for educational purposes only and not recommended as means of diagnosing or treating your specific condition. If you seek help, we encourage you to consult a physician and follow his or her professional advice.

Published by: Vermont Indie Books

Graphic design: Ediciones De La Parra

ISBN-13: 978-1514364802

ISBN-10: 1514364808

CONTENT

IN THE BEGINNING... THERE WAS MENOPAUSE!

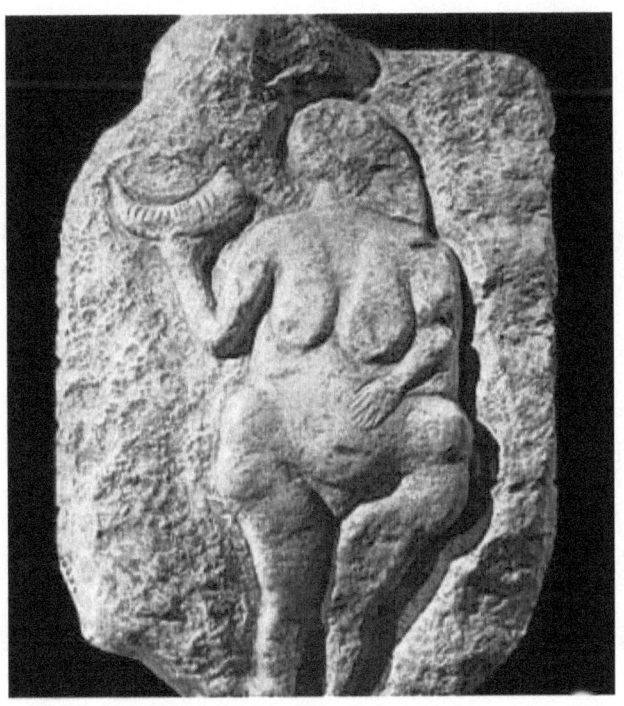

Berna Vermont

Menopause has been around since the dawn of the Stone Age, although back then and throughout all our ancient history, life expectancy was so low most men and women died in their childhood or youth, and only a small percentage made it to adulthood. To make things worse, maternal mortality was so high most females didn´t survive motherhood, and therefore only a minority experienced the symptoms of the different stages of menopause, a condition that was not properly studied - and much less understood- before the early 19th century.

Fact is, the word "menopause" was first coined in 1816, when the French physician Charles Pierre de Gardanne published a medical article called *"De la ménopause, ou de l'âge critique des femmes"* (*On menopause or the critical age of females*) in the pages of a prestigious French Journal. In his work, Gardanne first used the word *menespausie,* which he later shortened.

Gardanne described the condition as "a medical syndrome that affects women in the end of their fertile years". This was a hundred years before the isolation of estrogen, officially giving start to the long and winding quest for a definite "cure."

PIONEER STUDIES

The first medical textbook entirely dedicated to menopause was published over two decades later, in 1839, by the French physician C. F. Menville, who considered menopause a direct consequence of the natural "death of the womb", a description later adopted by most scientific specialists of his time and that in the early 20th century evolved and was popularized as the "the death of the woman in the woman."

The first major breakthrough came in the 1920s, when endocrinologists discovered insulin and, two years later, they identified and isolated estrogen found in ovarian follicular fluid. The following decade saw the birth of the first estrogen-like compounds and in 1940 the New York scientist Fuller Albright became the first to link osteoporosis to ovarian failure, coining the term "postmenopausal osteoporosis".

During the second half of the twentieth century and up to the early twenty-first century, most doctors prescribed hormone replacement therapy (HRT) to ease menopause symptoms. However, in 2002, the United States National Institutes of Health (NIH) showed that prolonged HRT actually boosts the risk of heart disease, stroke, breast cancer, and blood clots, causing more disease than it prevents. This is why an increasing number of doctors are now prescribing dietary supplements and herbal products together with a balanced diet, proper exercise and lifestyle changes.

THE PRESENT COMPILATION

This book is about how to cope with the different stages of menopause, its physical causes, basic symptoms and recommended treatments. It also includes priceless testimonials of women who've dealt with this condition, as well as selected facts and figures from recent studies conducted by leading scientists and specialists in the field.

I´d like to thank our collaborators: Elsa Markeys, Susy Mora, Mónica Parker and Daniel Parson, whose generous research and writings made this compilation possible and without whom it would never have seen public light.

MENOPAUSE: BASIC STAGES & SYMPTOMS

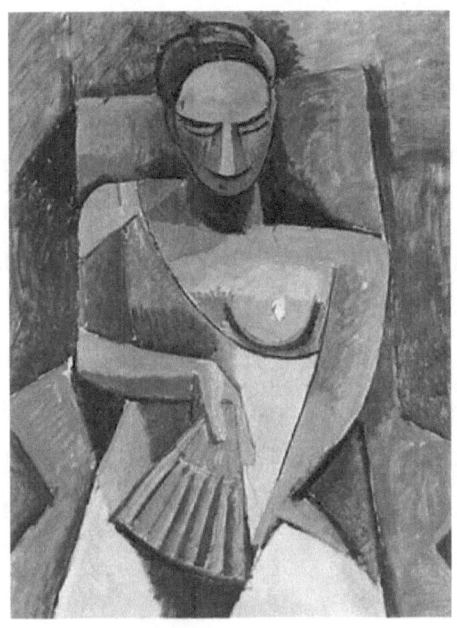

Berna Vermont

According to the National Institute on Aging (NIA), nearly 2 million U.S. women will turn 50 this year. And most of these females are experiencing or will experience the symptoms of perimenopause, menopause or post-menopause, three stages in a woman´s life bound to affect their physical and mental functions if not properly treated.

1:PERIMENOPAUSE:

Also known as "the prelude to menopause", this first stage generally begins when a woman is in her mid-forties, producing irregularities in the frequency, intensity and duration of her menstrual cycles and causing a series of unwanted physical and emotional symptoms that can last from 5 to 10 years.

Perimenopause begins with a drop in female hormone levels, changing the frequency, duration and intensity of a woman´s menstrual cycle which in spite of having been always regular, suddenly becomes unpredictable. Once she goes 12 months without menstruating, it is said that she has officially reached menopause. And, after this, she enters the stage of post-menopause, which will last the rest of her life and during which she may become prone to certain diseases, including bone loss (osteoporosis) and heart disease.

2:MENOPAUSE:

After going through the long years of perimenopause, in which a woman´s menstrual cycle become more and more infrequent, it is said that a woman officially reaches menopause once she has gone a full 12 months without menstruating (usually around 50 years of age).

3:POST-MENOPAUSE:

Once menopause has been reached a woman becomes permanently infertile and thus begins a new stage known as post-menopause, which will last for the rest of her life. Without proper treatment, during this last phase she may become prone to certain physical disorders, mainly bone loss (osteoporosis) and heart disease.

Although many women experience severe symptoms during their perimenopause, menopause and post-menopause, a small percentage of women pass these stages without experiencing any symptoms.

MOST FREQUENT SYMPTOMS:

Although some women go through these three stages without showing any symptoms, most experience at least one or more of the following:

HOT FLASHES: Scientifically known as vasomotor symptoms (VMS), they are experienced as a wave of intense heat that lasts from a couple of minutes to half an hour or more, producing sweating and faster heartbeat rates.

NIGHT SWEATS: Hot flashes during sleep produce what is known as "night sweats", usually interrupting sleep and causing insomnia and tiredness.

MOOD SWINGS: Sudden mood changes can be produced by fluctuations in hormone levels, as well as insomnia, night sweats, and anxiety.

IRRITABILITY: Hormonal fluctuations may also cause bad temper, popularly known as crankiness or "bitchy attitude" for no apparent reason.

BRAIN FOG: Described as memory loss and lack of concentration, this symptom threatens the productive lives of a vast percentage of women.

DEPPRESSION: Some women experience intense and recurring sadness for no apparent reason, mostly affecting those with a past history of depression.

LOSS OF SEX DRIVE: During menopause and post-menopause most women –not all- experience vaginal dryness and a lack of sexual desire.

INSOMNIA: Sleep disorder is generally produced by other menopause symptoms, such as night sweats, headaches, depression and anxiety.

ANXIETY: Drops in hormone levels and the inability to cope with aging and change produce in some women "anxiety attacks" for no apparent reason.

HEADACHES: Hormone drops can cause headaches or menstrual migraines in women who reach perimenopause -even if they´ve never had them.

More details about these symptoms and how to fight them in the following chapters.

HOW I FACED "THE YEARS OF CHANGE"

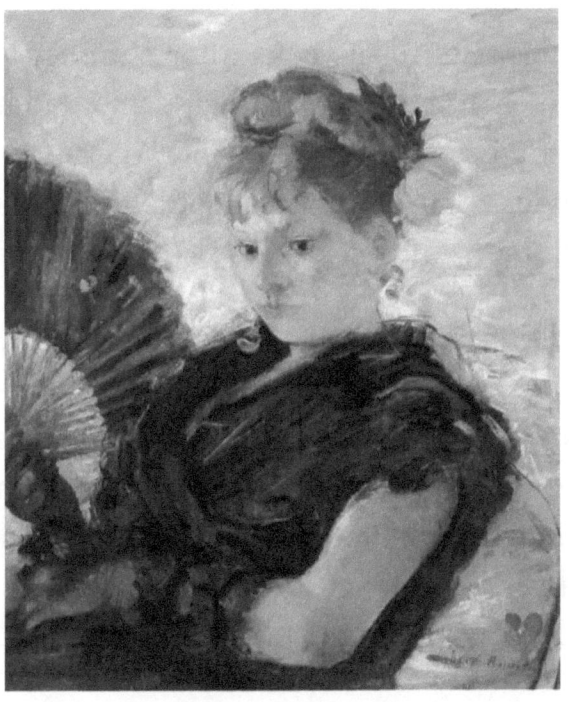

Elsa Markeys

I'm a 57-year old retired schoolteacher and a proud mother of two lovely young women who have given me five grandsons. After dealing with perimenopause and menopause, popularly known as "The Change" I wish to share my experience in this site.

I'm presently in my post-menopause years and God knows getting old hasn't been easy. I was 46 years old when I missed my period for two months. This had only happened to me when I'd been pregnant, but this time I was divorced and had been living like a secluded nun for almost a year.

To my surprise, four weeks after I missed my second period, I menstruated twice that same month! That's when I started getting my first hot flashes and sudden mood changes. I knew then that something was changing deep within me.

After putting it off for some weeks, I finally went to see doctor Robert E.Thompson, who ran some tests and. before I knew it, he gave me the news: I had reached my perimenopause, as most women do in their mid-forties. It's a period in life that precedes menopause, usually lasting between 5 and 10 years and mistakenly called pre-menopause by many. I was deeply shocked.

I had always dreaded menopause. Why? Because ever since I had my first period, back when I was thirteen, my mother told me about the different stages of womanhood, from the fertile years to menopause. I dreaded its very name!

I had always believed that menopause would mean the end of my sexual life as well as my productive years. I was so wrong!

As my doctor explained, during perimenopause the levels of the hormones estrogen and progestin begins to drop, affecting women both physically and mentally. These hormones are vital for women in their fertile years and a drop in their levels produces irregular periods with shorter, longer, heavier or lighter cycles, ultimately leading to the cessation of menstruation and producing dramatic long-term consequences.

He also said these hormones can be taken artificially to ease perimenopausal and menopausal symptoms, a medical practice known as Hormone Replacement Therapy or HRT. However, in 2003 the Women's Health Initiative (WHI) published a study highlighting the dangers of extended use of HRT, which can actually boost the risk of breast cancer and heart disease in women with tendencies for those diseases in their family and medical backgrounds. And since my mother had had breast cancer and her father (my grandfather) had died of heart disease, I immediately realized that HRT was out of the question.

Shortly after I started my treatment, which consisted in a balanced diet, daily exercise and natural supplements, mainly vitamins, minerals and herbal products proven to alleviate symptoms, like soy (soybeans, tofu, and soymilk), ginseng, chromium, niacin, black cohosh, red clover, chaste-berry, wild yam, red raspberry, grape seed, ginger and damiana, among others. I also found that estrogen creams can reduce certain specific symptoms without the unwanted consequences generated by HRT and presently I feel better than ever!

MY EXPERIENCE WITH HOT FLASHES

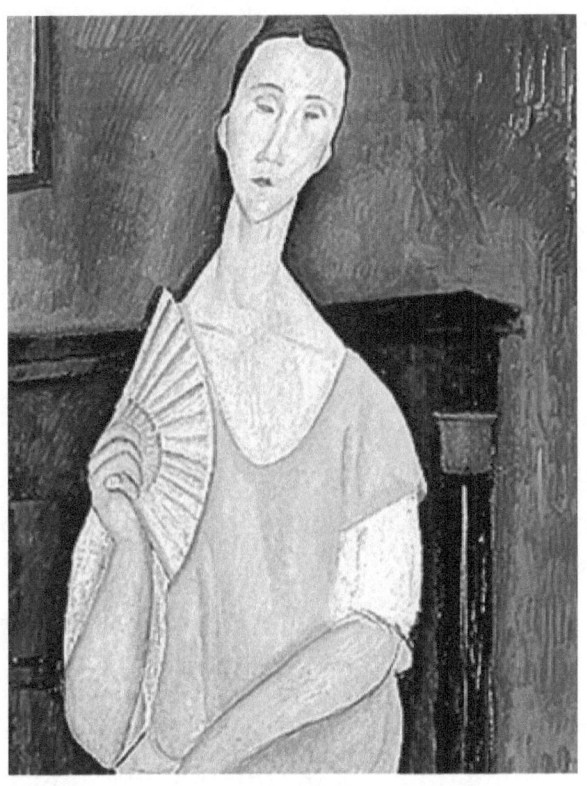

Susy Mora

Based on my own experience, hot flashes are one of the most uncomfortable symptoms ever experienced by women in their perimenopause and menopause years.

Although hot flashes are sometimes bearable, occasionally they can be so intense to seriously affect your daily routine. I was 47 when I first experienced them and I first thought I was ill. Back then I had no idea about the symptoms of menopause nor that I was actually in my first year of perimenopause. And when the truth finally surfaced I started reading all I could about my new "condition" as well as the best and most effective ways to fight its main symptoms.

I'd like to share my *Basic Facts About Hot Flashes*, based on my own experience and all the information I've gathered since I first experienced them:

• A hot flash is like a wave of sudden fever spreading through the body, usually affecting the head and neck regions and causing immediate perspiration and flushing.
• Although it is believed that hot flashes are the effect of decreasing estrogen levels, to this date scientists still haven't found its true physical causes.
• Most women facing perimenopause and menopause experience recurring hot flashes (up to 80% in their fifth year and down to 10% ten years after reaching menopause)
• They often come at night, interrupting sleep and causing night sweats, insomnia and daytime tiredness.
• They come in different intensities and generally last from brief seconds to a few minutes.

• They affect women as well as their bed partners, generating sleep deprivation and causing daytime tiredness in both partners.

• According to a Cochrane Prospective Meta-Analysis (PMA), oral hormone therapy (estrogens only or estrogens with progesterone) is highly effective in diminishing hot flashes. Nevertheless, with the declining use of hormone replacement therapy, natural products have recently become the best alternative for women seeking to decrease the recurrence and intensity of hot flashes in a safe and healthy way.

SLEEP DISORDER: GETTING THROUGH THE NIGHT

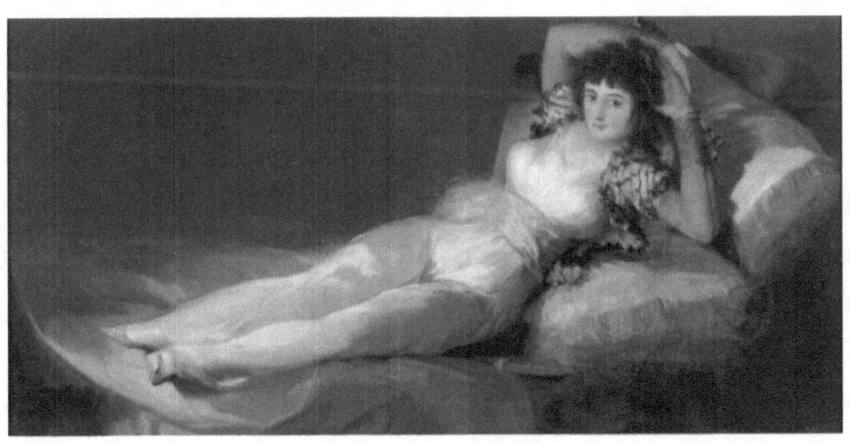

Daniel Parson

One of the most uncomfortable symptoms that affect women as they approach menopause is sleep disorder. According to the National Sleep Foundation, approximately 61% of menopausal and post-menopausal women experience sleep problems at least several nights a week. In women between the ages of 35 and 55, according to research, this disorder affects over half of the female population. And it also tends to increase with age if not treated properly.

Also known as "insomnia" and "sleeplessness", this condition is generally described as *"the impossibility of falling or staying asleep"*. And, even though it affects women at night, sleeping difficulties can produce severe daytime consequences, including sleepiness, drowsiness, memory loss, lack of concentration, irritability, and mood changes, among other symptoms, thus affecting her daily life.

Despite the fact that sleep disorders is usually associated with a drop in female hormone levels (mainly estrogen and progesterone), this condition is really the direct consequence of other symptoms of perimenopause, menopause and post-menopause, mainly hot flashes and night sweat, which are experienced by approximately 80% of menopausal women. Other well-known causes for sleep disorder in these women are anxiety attacks, states of depression, and pauses or gasps in breathing during sleep (apnea).

Apart from sleeping pills, there are several alternative treatments worth mentioning. The most recommended are natural products and supplements that include calcium, vitamin D, bisphosphonates. Also recommended are soy products (tofu, soybeans, and soymilk), which contain a plant-hormone similar to estrogen (phytoestrogen); ginseng biloba, as well as red clover and black cohosh extracts, among others.

If you are experiencing difficulties in falling or staying asleep due to hot flashes and night sweat, keep your room cool and well ventilated at nights and try to wear loose clothing to bed –a natural fiber like cotton is recommended. Also recommended is going to bed at the same time each night, according to a regular bedtime schedule. And, before going to bed, avoid excessive caffeine and spicy foods that tend to cause sweating. In any case, if you want to ease these symptoms and improve your sleep, ask your doctor about the benefits of natural supplements and how they can help you regain a normal life.

HOW I LOST MY JOB DUE TO MENOPAUSE

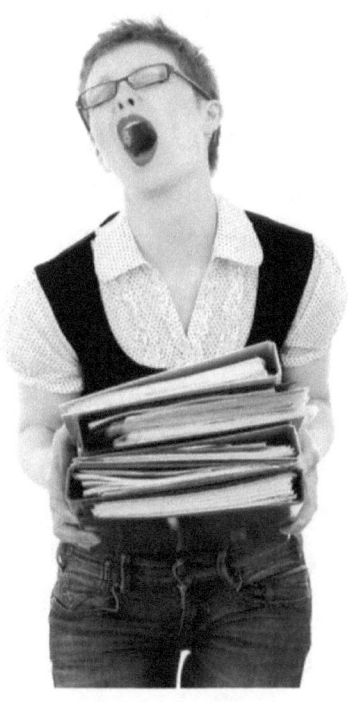

Monica Parker

A couple of years ago I lost my job due to one of the most dreadful symptoms that has affected me during my first years of perimenopause. Known as "brain fog", it's a mental state that affects a wide number of women in their late 40s and in their 50s, diminishing their intellectual performance and therefore jeopardizing their jobs and professional careers, as happened in my case.

Back then I was the creative director of a medium-sized advertising agency and didn't know that my "mental problem" was a symptom of perimenopause and that it could easily be treated. If only I had known then what I know today!

It's like a "sudden lapsus", a temporary memory loss or incapability to concentrate. Based on my experience, somewhat s comparable to the Tip-of-the-tongue state (TOT), the feeling you get when you can't remember something you're sure you know, while sensing that you "almost have it" and that it's "on the tip of your tongue".

A real bummer, that's what it is! Especially for successful working women like me! It took me ten years to reach one of the agency's top positions and only a couple to ruin it all. Just imagine being in the middle of an important presentation or meeting and suddenly forgetting your client's name or what you're talking about. Or spending hours writing a piece of advertising or developing a creative strategy and forgetting what you're doing an instant before someone asks you something important about your work. Once I even flew to a different state to meet with an important client and after I got there I realized I'd left my laptop with the presentation back at the office! And when the client greeted me I didn't remember his name and didn't even know what I was doing there!

Of course, these states were only temporary, and not always as intense. The worst cases, like the ones I just mentioned, were rather infrequent and I must say that most of the time I was fit for work. But when your intellectual skills are needed on a daily basis -as in the case of a creative director in charge of a dozen accounts and managing a team of copywriters and art directors, like me- after two years I was unable to hide my flaws. Finally, due to my recurring "lapsus" our advertising agency lost its two most important clients and I was forced to resign.

Luckily, I now know that "brain fog" is treatable and, thanks to my doctor, I followed a 100% natural treatment that not only "unfogged" my mind but also diminished all my other perimenopause symptoms.

Last December, as a happy corollary, I opened a small advertising agency with an ex-coworker and we soon got a couple of important clients, so I´m doing great! In sum, thanks to natural therapy, the brain fog is gone and I´m surging the fast-lane to success!

Coping With Menopause

BRAIN FOG: BASIC FACTS & TREATMENTS

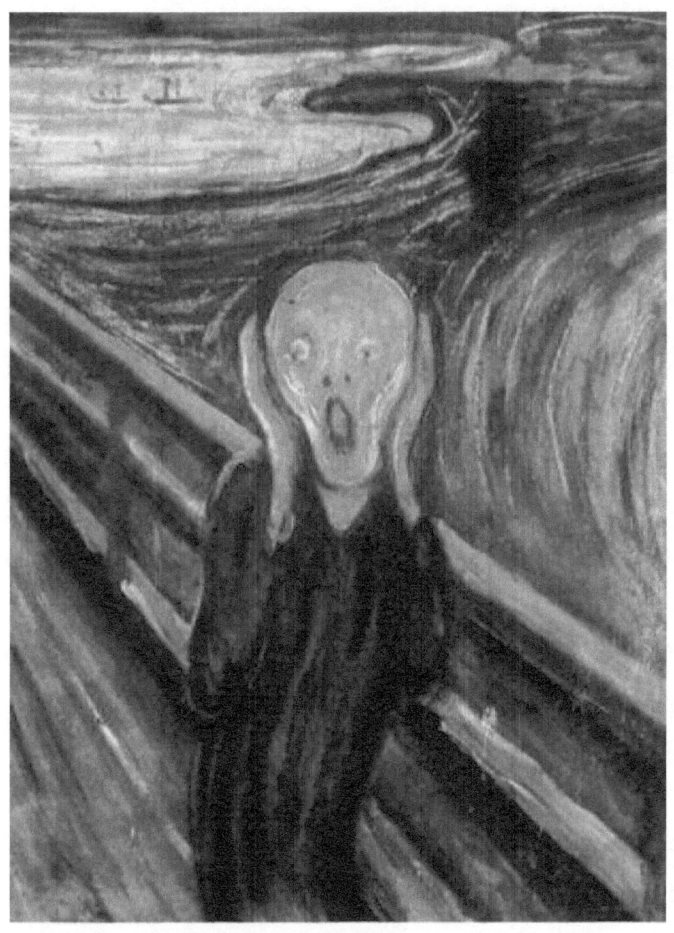

Monica Parker

Millions of female workers in their late 40s and in their 50s have experienced "brain fog", bouts of forgetfulness or lack of concentration that are presently being studied by an increasing number of scientists throughout the world in hope of understanding the hidden process that lies within the brain as women approach the age of menopause.

To better understand the cognitive changes that take place during this phase in a female's life, a group of scientists at the University of Rochester Medical Center and the University of Illinois at Chicago recently studied a group of 75 women in their perimenopause or menopause years (ages 40 to 60). The study was led by the University of Rochester Medical Center neuropsychologist Miriam Weber, Ph.D., who explained that the voluntaries were given a series of cognitive tests to measure their learning and memory skills, as well as their concentration and problem-solving capability. The study showed that only certain percentage of women (from one-third to two-thirds) evidenced some type of memory or concentration problems and that most of these also reported symptoms of depression, anxiety, and sleep difficulties.

Regarding the best natural ways to relieve brain fog, a growing number of scientists believe that key is adequate nutrition, including sufficient nutrients, minerals and omega-3 fatty acids, which can be taken as natural supplements, as well as multivitamins and vitamin B12.

Among the herbal remedies and supplements proven to relief brain fog is gingko biloba, a millenary herb extracted from the leaves of the ginkgo tree. It has been used in China for over 5,000 years and is known to boost circulation and enhance brain functions by dilating blood vessels and increasing oxygen flow in neural tissue.

In recent decades prestigious studies have proven that gingko biloba improves cognitive functions and memory, boosting the brain's capability to fact retention, communicate ideas, memory retrieval and problem solving. It has no known side-effects and can be safely taken with other supplements. Apart from increasing the brain's oxygen flow, recent biochemical tests have also showed that it inhibits toxins in the brain and EEG tracings have evidenced its capacity to stimulate brain wave activity.

FEMALE WORKERS AND MENOPAUSE

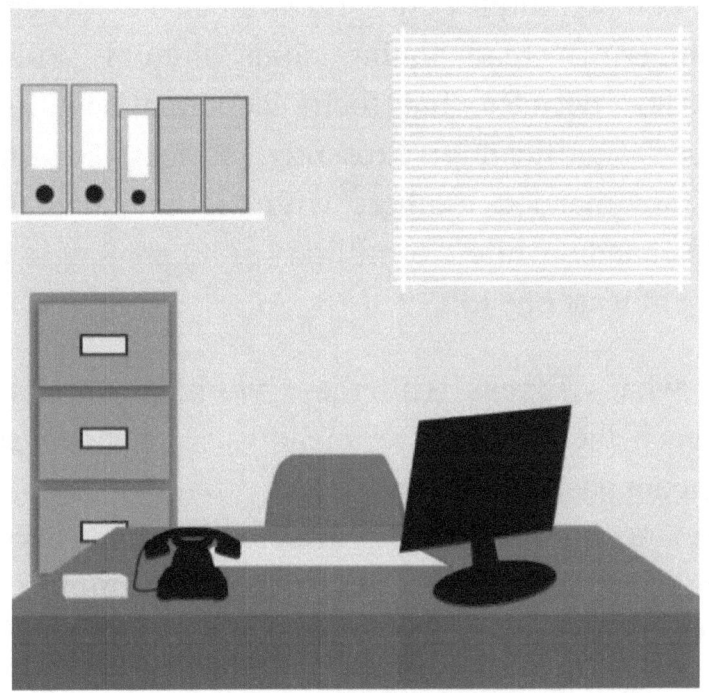

Daniel Parson

According to a 2013 study based on U.S. Census Bureau figures and conducted by the Pew Research Center, 40% of all households with children under the age of 18 in the United States are led by women as sole or primary providers. This represents a 29% increase from 1960, when these were only 11%.

In fact, according to the U.S. Federal Interagency Forum on Child and Family Statistics, the number of American homes led by women is not only growing at steady pace, but it is actually eight times higher than those led by single fathers.

The Pew Research Center research also evidenced that the number of "breadwinning moms" not only multiplied in the last decades, but their economic benefits also increased significantly: Presently, at least 5.1 million (37%) are married mothers with higher incomes than their husbands, while 8.6 million (63%) are single moms holding at least one job.

But what happens with these working women once they reach the years of perimenopause, menopause and post-menopause? Is it true that, in most cases, their performance is negatively affected by the hormonal changes that alter their bodily functions during these years?

Truth is, a significant percentage of these women not only experience a noticeable drop in their concentration and memory levels, but also experience sudden hot flashes in their work, drowsiness due to lack of sleep at night, sudden mood changes, anxiety attacks, and states of depression and irritability. They begin to feel that, as working women, they are starting to "lose it" and are suddenly troubled by the fear of losing their productive working life for good.

Although a small percentage of women never experience these symptoms, a significant number are directly affected. However, recent studies have ratified the effectiveness of natural supplements in diminishing these symptoms, allowing women to prolong their active, working lives without the unwanted consequences of aging. If you are experiencing these symptoms, take your time to learn all you can about the many benefits of natural-products therapy and please consult your local physician!

SEXUAL DESIRE DURING "THE CHANGE"

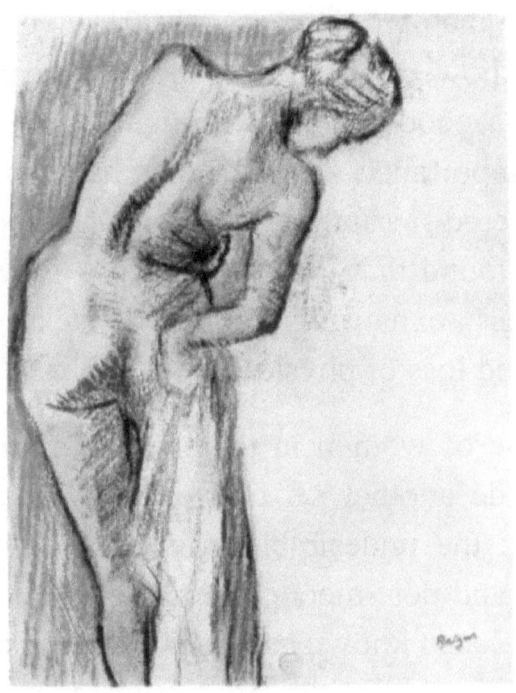

Elsa Markeys

Reaching menopause is like a sexual "Russian roulette" for women. Why? Because a wide number of them are destined to experience an important drop in their sexual drive, including decreased pleasure with penetration, difficulty reaching climax, weak orgasmic sensations or pain during sex. The good news is that a small percentage of these women experience no change whatsoever and some even experience an increase in their sexual desire!

For most married women, marital sex is vital to keep a relationship alive. This view was the basis of a recent survey conducted by the online women's community iVillage with the participation of 1,001 wives ages 18-49. The survey showed that 75% of the participants admitted that sharing a good sex life with their couple is "very or extremely important". On the other hand, only 16% of them considered marital sex "somewhat important." The survey also found that the main reasons for not wanting sex are stress, exhaustion, children, lack of romance, arguments and loss of physical attraction.

In the case of women in their mid-40s and older, we should include another set of important reasons for not wanting sex: the undesirable effects of perimenopause, menopause, and post-menopause. These three stages in a woman´s life, also known as "The Change", are produced from a natural drop in the production of hormones like estrogen and progesterone, which regulate fertility, menstruation, procreation and maternity, therefore affecting a wide number of bodily functions.

Pain during intercourse seems to be the main reason for most of women who lose interest in sex during "The Change". This pain is generally caused by vaginal dryness (derived from thinner vaginal lining), causing difficulties and maltreatment during sexual intercourse.

Researchers have found conflicting results regarding estrogen replacement therapy as a treatment for vaginal dryness. In turn, most doctor recommend the use of lubricants (like K-Y jelly, for example) as well as estrogen creams, which lubricate and restore the lining's thickness and consistency when applied vaginally.

During "The Change", it must be said, sexual performance can also be affected by hot flashes, night sweats, brain fog, mood swings, irritability, depression, and headaches, among others. If you are experiencing some or all of these symptoms, my advice is to wake up and take a stand. Find out all you can about the different therapies available and please consult your physician!

MENOPAUSE & ANDROPAUSE

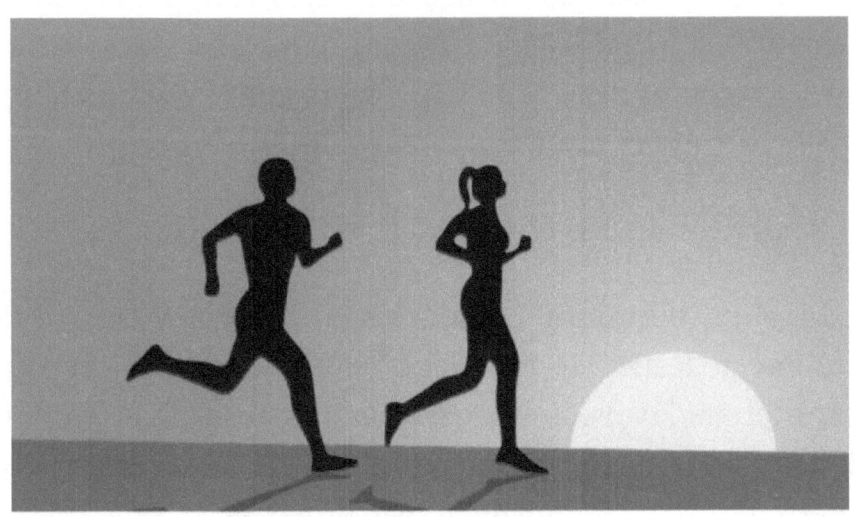

Monica Parker

What causes menopause? And is it true that men also experience a similar stage known as andropause?

Menopause, as well as andropause, are both natural consequences of aging. In the case of women it begins with a 5 to 10 year period known as perimenopause, which generally occurs around the age of 45.

Statistics evidence that the age of perimenopause and menopause may vary from one person to another and is determined in large part by the female's hereditary background, as well as her nutrition and health habits, including smoking (which is known to accelerate the process).

Premature menopause takes place before age 40 in 8 percent of women and is also known as early menopause, generally induced by the surgical removal of the ovaries (hysterectomy) or due to damages produced by chemotherapy or radiation therapy.

ANDROPAUSE OR MALE MENOPAUSE

In men, the aging-related stage in which there is a decline in testicular functions, and therefore a drop in testosterone levels, is known as andropause. This is often defined as "male menopause" and is alternatively referred to as hypogonadism. Nevertheless, it only affects a small percentage of men and usually begins at age 40.

Unlike menopause in women, andropause takes place even more gradually, with testosterone levels decreasing over the course of decades. Normal symptoms include decreased libido, mood changes, depression and erectile dysfunction.

In any case, both menopause and andropause are natural processes that can be medically treated. If you believe you're experiencing any of the two, my honest advice is to consult your physician. Remember that these lines are for educational purposes only and not recommended as a means of diagnosing or treating your specific condition.

RECOMMENDED TREATMENTS

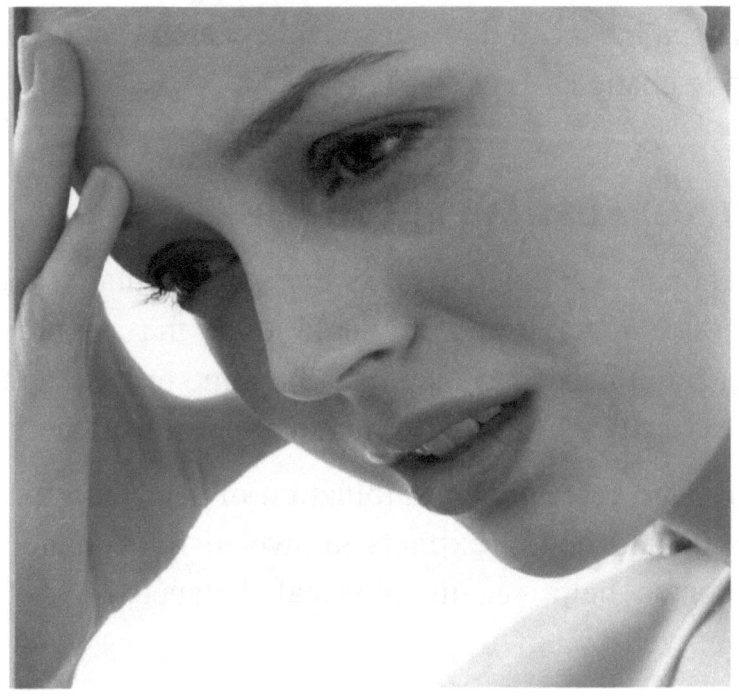

Berna Vermont

Despite the fact that for over half a century hormone replacement therapy (HRT) was generally used to fight menopause symptoms, as I explained in the first chapter of this book, in 2002 the U. S. National Institute of Health (NIH) evidenced that an important percentage of women are negatively affected by this practice, proven to actually increase the risk of heart disease, stroke, breast cancer, and blood clots. Jesus! Just think of the thousands of women who took this therapy over the last decades and died due to this unprecedented "medical error"! This is why most doctors presently focus on 100% natural treatments that have proven to be effective and without side effects, including dietary supplements, herbal extracts, a balanced diet, reasonable exercise, and healthy lifestyle changes.

MENOPAUSE SUPPLEMENTS

Menopause supplements, as they are popularly known, are 100% natural and are sold over the counter (no prescription needed). They usually come in pill form and have no artificial hormones nor adverse side effects.

They are basically a combination of selected vitamins, minerals and herbal extracts known to fight menopause symptoms, help regain physical balance, and boost general well-being:

Among the most recommended are *Femestron, Estropin, Amberen,* and *Estroven,* which include safe and effective natural ingredients that have been scientifically proven to relieve menopause symptoms, such as chromium, niacin, black cohosh, red clover, chasteberry, soybean isoflavones.

Chromium, for example, is commonly found in processed meats, coffee, tea, potatoes, peas, oysters, cereals, brewer's yeast, rye, thyme, whole grains, and beer. It is helpful in treating brain fog, reduces risks of heart disease, and regulates the metabolism of sugar and fat.

Niacin, on the other hand, is also known as vitamin B3 and participates in over 50 metabolic processes, including the production of sex hormones.

Also known to fight the main menopause symptoms are soybeans, which have a high content of isoflavones and are rich in antioxidants, omega-3's, and protein, helping to reduce hot flashes, night sweats, irritability, mood changes, headaches, restore bone bone growth, improve heart health, and reduce weight.

Other ingredients you should look for when buying a menopause supplements are black cohosh, chaste berry and red clover, which have proven to help restore hormonal balance and reduce hot flashes, night sweats, and anxiety, among other symptoms.

IMPORTANCE OF A HEALTHY DIET

According to the British Dietetic Association (BDA), along with menopause supplements, a healthy, balanced diet is also necessary to combat the unwanted symptoms of perimenopause, menopause and post-menopause. Truth is, most doctors now emphasize the importance of eating certain nutriments, along with exercising and healthy lifestyle changes.

The following tips are most useful when planning a healthy diet:

- Always grill instead of frying your food.

•Make sure to drink only semi-skimmed, 1% or skimmed milk.

•Always opt for low or reduced-fat dairy products.

•Cut down on salt and avoid processed foods.

•Always eat plenty of fruits and vegetables, as well as oats, wholegrain cereals and beans.

•Vitamin D is very important and is found in cereals, eggs, red meat, oily fish, cod liver oil, and fortified margarine, among other foods.

•Regarding the loss of calcium that affects women as they approach menopause, causing osteoporosis, scientists have found that many natural nutrients can help to maintain healthy calcium levels, including fruit and vegetables as well as foods from the milk and dairy group, for these provide calcium. Also a must are calcium supplements.

•Due to the fact that during menopause and post-menopause the risk of heart disease may increase, your diet should include less saturated and trans fats and more lean cuts of meat, without excess fat, avoiding processed meat products.

•Keep away from sodas and junk food (including fast-food). A healthy diet will help you prevent the weight gain triggered during the perimenopause and menopause, when most women lose muscle mass and therefore their bodies need less calories to survive.

•See a specialist. Remember that this book is for educational purposes only and is not recommended as a means of diagnosing or treating your specific condition. If you are experiencing perimenopause, menopause, or post-menopause symptoms and need treatment and a healthy diet planned especially for your particular case, please consult your physician or nutritionist.

THANKS FOR READING THIS BOOK!

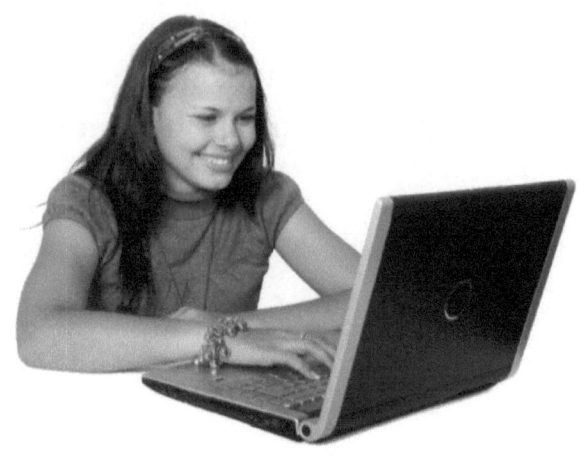

If you found this book helpful, please consider taking a few moments to leave your REVIEW on Amazon!

GO TO AMAZON BOOKPAGE

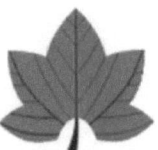

Vermont Indie Books

2015

OTHER BOOKS BY BERNA VERMONT

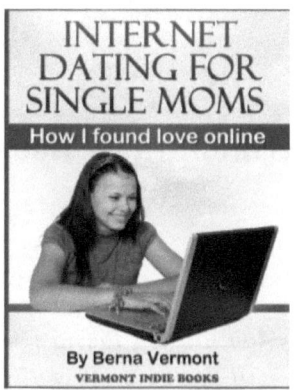

SEE DETAILS IN AMAZON.COM

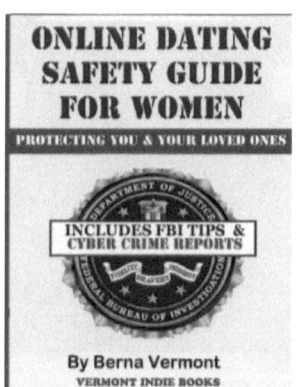

SEE DETAILS IN AMAZON.COM

PUBLISHED BY:

Vermont Indie Books
2015